ULTIMATE AID

TO

MY PREGNANCY JOURNEY

SANDRA W.PARKER

TABLE OF CONTENT

Contents

INTRODUCTION

It's important to get ready for pregnancy before you start your adventure. You should be aware that a pregnancy is a 40-week journey into motherhood, beginning at conception and ending at delivery. Beginning on the first day of your last menstrual period (LMP), you and your unborn child will encounter new milestones every trimester, including physical changes, changing pregnancy symptoms, and an increase in the size of the fetus. To discuss your plans and make sure you are in good health, see your healthcare professional. Examine your home for any possible risks or changes that need to be made. Make lifestyle adjustments, such as giving up alcohol and smoking, as these can negatively impact both your fertility and the health of your unborn child. To guarantee that you have sufficient amounts of vital nutrients like folic acid, iron, and calcium, it would be ideal if you also thought about taking prenatal[1] vitamins. Work with your healthcare practitioner to properly manage any pre-existing health issues, such as diabetes or hypertension, before becoming pregnant.

CHAPTER 1
THE FIRST TRIMESTER

Although becoming a parent is an exciting and fulfilling experience, you probably have a lot of questions and sometimes feel overwhelmed. That's normal, and we hope this information will help you along the way while you become pregnant. Both your body and your unborn child are growing and changing during the first 13 weeks of pregnancy. This is what you should know when you begin your incredible journey together.

WHAT ARE YOU FEELING?

Your body is about to go through a significant transition as it gets ready to grow a new life.

Missed periods are the first indication of pregnancy in women with regular monthly menstrual cycles. Bleeding during implantation can happen occasionally. This bleeding resembles a mild period or spotting quite a bit. Even though this is quite normal, if you suffer any bleeding during your pregnancy, you should consult your healthcare professional.

You can begin to feel tired or queasy, or you might discover that you have more energy than usual! Pay attention to your body and modify your workouts as necessary. Every pregnancy is unique, just like every woman. Moreover, a few of the symptoms listed below, such exhaustion, nausea, or more frequent urination, may appear early in your pregnancy.

MORE REGULAR SYMPTOMS

Your entire body is impacted by the hormonal changes that occur during the first few weeks of pregnancy. Although every pregnancy is unique, the following symptoms can arise in the first trimester:

Breast tenderness; severe mood swings; nausea or vomiting (morning sickness); frequent urination; weight gain or loss;

extreme exhaustion; headaches; heartburn; leg cramps; lower back and pelvic discomfort; changing food cravings into new dislikes; constipation

TREATING ONESELF FOR THE SYMPTOMS

To put it mildly, early pregnancy symptoms can be quite painful. After seeing your healthcare physician, try these techniques for some alleviation. Never forget that decisions should always be based on your tastes and the resources at your disposal.

• Ginger, chamomile, vitamin B6, and/or acupuncture can help with nausea and vomiting.

• Try calcium or magnesium for leg cramps.

•If the dietary changes recommended by your healthcare physician are not alleviating your constipation, you may consider using wheat bran or other fiber supplements.

Throughout your whole pregnancy, it's crucial to eat a healthy diet and get frequent exercise. Maintain your regular exercise regimen for as long as it makes you feel comfortable. It will be simpler for you to adjust to your changing physique if you maintain an active lifestyle during your pregnancy. Make sure to feed your developing body and the growing body of your infant healthy foods. By consuming a range of nutritious foods, such as fruits, vegetables, meat, beans, nuts, pasteurized dairy, and veggies, you may ensure that you are getting enough energy, protein, vitamins, and minerals.

HOW YOUR CHILD IS DEVELOPING

The most important time for your baby's development is during this phase. Your baby's physique and internal systems are starting to take shape during the first trimester. The following early organ and body developments are listed:

- Kidneys

- Liver

- Eyes

- Genitalia

- Inner ear

- Cardiac tissue

- Brain and spine

- Fingernails

- A pancreas; and so on.

- Lungs;

- Mouth, eye, and nose muscles

- Webbed fingers and toes

- Hands, feet, and limb cartilage

For a variety of reasons, fetal growth can vary greatly; nonetheless, in the first trimester, your baby's measurements will increase from less than a grain of rice at the end of the first month to approximately 10 cm (4 in) by the end of week 12, weighing approximately 28 g.

CHAPTER 2

THE SECOND TRIMESTER

Your second trimester is upon you! In comparison to the first trimester, many women discover that they experience fewer symptoms. When your womb develops larger and more vertical at this stage of your pregnancy, you could notice a little baby bump.

EMOTIONS YOU ARE FEELING

Although each woman's experience is unique, many expectant mothers report feeling better in the second trimester than in the first. With luck, you'll begin to experience less weariness and nausea.

When your pregnancy reaches the third trimester, you should feel your unborn child move and kick! You will also notice some new changes, such as a developing tummy.

MORE REGULAR SYMPTOMS

Although every pregnancy is unique, the following symptoms can occur in the second trimester:

• The sensation of tingling, numbness, or weakness in your hands caused by carpal tunnel syndrome

• A crease that extends from your belly button to your pubic hairline

• Darker patches on your face;

• Reduced pelvic and back pain;

• Darkening areola;

• Stretch marks on your thighs, buttocks, belly, and breasts.

TREATING ONESELF FOR THE SYMPTOMS

During the second trimester, you should start to see larger changes in your body even if your symptoms should be lessening. After consulting your healthcare physician, consider some of the following techniques to help relieve some of the aches and pains that may accompany these changes. Never forget that decisions should always be based on your tastes and the resources at your disposal.

• It is advised to exercise regularly throughout pregnancy to help with pelvic and lower back pain. Numerous alternative treatment modalities, including acupuncture, support belts, and physiotherapy, can also be employed.

• To treat carpal tunnel syndrome, elevate your wrist and hand, rest, and apply ice.

• If you want to apply a cream, gel, or lotion for stretch marks, apply it as soon as possible and massage it into the markings. Using the selected product every day for several weeks at a time is also crucial.

Throughout your pregnancy, especially in the second trimester, eating well and exercising frequently are essential. Continue your regular exercise regimen, but don't overdo it. You should be able to carry on a conversation while exercising, generally speaking. Always get advice from your doctor before exercising while pregnant. To ensure that you are getting enough protein, vitamins, minerals, and energy, keep consuming a variety of meals.

THE WAY YOUR CHILD IS GROWING

Throughout the second trimester, the internal organs and biological processes of your unborn child are developing in an increasingly intricate way. These crucial weeks see the full development of the brain's motor control center, the hardening of bones, the formation of thick skin and toenails, the beginning of the nervous system and hearing, the opening and closing of the eyelids, the strengthening of the kicks, the functioning of the digestive system, and the full development of the lungs.

Your baby will be about 10 cm (4 in) and weigh about 28 g (1 oz) at the start of the second trimester, however fetal growth can vary greatly for a variety of reasons. Your developing child will weigh between 1 and 2 kg (2 and 4 pounds) and be around 35 cm (14 in) long by the time your second trimester concludes.

CHAPTER 3

THE THIRD TRIMESTER

Congratulations, you've made it to the finish line! A stunning new family member will soon be joining you. Even if these past several weeks have been more difficult and exhausting for you, you still have a lot to look forward to!

WHAT ARE YOU FEELING?

You'll still experience some of the same discomforts from your second trimester. In addition, a lot of women experience difficulty breathing and notice that they need to use the restroom more frequently. This is a result of your organs being under increased strain from the growing baby. Rest assured, your baby is doing well, and these issues will runaway once you give birth.

TYPICAL   SIGNS   AND   SYMPTOMS

While every pregnancy is unique, the following symptoms can occur in the third trimester:

Acid reflux (heartburn)

- Hemorrhoids

- Breathlessness

- Tenderness in the breasts

- Difficulty falling asleep

- Swelling in the fingers, face, and ankles

SELF-CARE TO ALLEVIATE SYMPTOMS

You can feel more discomfort in the third trimester than in the second because your baby is getting closer to full term. After seeing your healthcare practitioner, try some of the following techniques to alleviate some of the agony. Never forget that decisions should always be based on your tastes and the resources at your disposal.

• Consult your doctor for guidance on food and lifestyle changes if you have heartburn. For more problematic symptoms, antacid medications can be employed if they don't work.

• If you have trouble falling asleep, consider using a pillow to support your entire body or just the troublesome areas. It will assist release tension while you sleep.

• Eating well and exercising frequently are crucial throughout the third trimester of pregnancy. Continue your regular exercise regimen, but don't overdo it. You should be able to carry on a conversation while exercising, generally speaking. Always get advice from your doctor before exercising while pregnant.

You'll still experience some of the same discomforts from your second trimester. In addition, a lot of women experience difficulty breathing and notice that they need to use the restroom more frequently. This is a result of your organs being under increased strain from the growing baby. Rest assured, your baby is doing well, and these issues will go away once you give birth.

- BRAXTON HICKS (FALSE CONTRACTIONS)

You will also have contractions in the third trimester, which may indicate either false or actual labor. Braxton Hicks pains, sometimes known as **"false labor,"** are your body's method of getting ready for real labor. They could have an abdominal tightening or menstrual cramping sensation. Braxton Hicks does not have a medical cure, however there are certain things you can do to lessen discomfort, such as:

• Sipping water;

- Switching positions (walking is a good idea if you're lying down);

- Napping;

- Reading a book;

- Or soothing music;

If none of these help, or if you start to notice an increase in the frequency or intensity of your contractions, see a doctor.

HOW YOUR BABY IS GROWING

During this final stage of development, your little one is getting ready to leave the womb. Between the beginning of the third trimester and birth:

- Eyes can sense changes in light
- Head might have some hair
- Can kick, grasp and stretch
- Limbs begin to look chubby
- Bones harden
- Circulatory system is complete
- Musculoskeletal system is complete
- Lungs, brain and nervous system are developed
- Fat continues to be added

Fetal growth can vary significantly for a number of reasons, but at the beginning of the third trimester, your baby will be around 35 cm (4 in) long and weigh from 1 to 2 kg (2 to 4 lbs). By the time you give birth, your newborn will be about 46 to 51 cm (18 to 20 in) long and weigh just over 3 kg (7 lbs) .

STARTING   A   LABOUR

It's common for women to give birth between 38 and 41 weeks of pregnancy, but it's impossible to predict when labor will start. The cervix dilates and the uterine muscles start to contract at regular intervals, gradually drawing closer together as labor progresses. Menstrual cramps and contractions will feel alike, but contractions will be stronger. Your abdomen will harden and you may experience back or pelvic pain when your uterus contracts. Your belly will soften again as your uterus relaxes.

Other indications that labor is starting besides contractions are:

• Lightening (the feeling that the fetus has lowered)

• Mucus plug loss (more clear or pink discharge will be visible).

• Water breaking (membrane rupture)

It's crucial to remember that some of these changes could go unnoticed before labor starts. Get in touch with your healthcare professional if you believe you are in labor.

CHAPTER 4

FOOD TO EAT WHEN PREGNANT

Maintaining a nutritious diet is vital at any stage of life, but it becomes even more crucial while you are expecting. Your baby will grow, develop, and maintain a healthy weight with the support of a balanced diet.

WHICH DIET SHOULD I FOLLOW DURING PREGNANCY? A diet rich in nutrients consists of a range of wholesome items from every food category.

FRUIT

Dried, frozen, or fresh fruit are all excellent options. Fruits and vegetables should make up half of your plate at mealtimes.

VEGETABLE

Vegetables can be eaten frozen, tinned, or uncooked. Dark leafy greens are a healthy option for salads. Fruits and vegetables should make up half of your plate at mealtimes.

GRAINS

Make half of your grain servings at mealtimes whole grains. Unprocessed grains, such as whole grains, contain the entire grain kernel. Oats, barley, quinoa, brown rice, and bulgur are a few examples.

PROTEIN

Eating different types of proteins every day is vital. Foods high in protein include meat, poultry, beans, peas, eggs, almonds, and seeds.

DIARY

Make sure the dairy products you choose have undergone pasteurization. Milk and dairy products like cheese and plain yogurt are healthy choices.

FATS AND OILS

Limit your intake of solid fats, such as duck fat or other fats derived from animals. Other foods, such some fish, avocados, and nuts, have healthier fats. The majority of the oils in food are derived from plants (such canola and olive oils).

MINERAL AND VITAMIN REQUIRED BY PREGNANT WOMAN

Throughout your pregnancy, you should make sure you're obtaining the following essential vitamins and minerals:

CALCIUM

Aim for 1,000 mg of calcium every day to help your baby's teeth and bones grow. Dark green leafy vegetables, milk, cheese, and plain yogurt are a few excellent sources.

IRON

Aim for 27 mg/day of iron. Iron aids in the delivery of oxygen to your developing child through red blood cells. It's accessible to you.

Lean red meat, chicken, peas, and beans are good sources of it.

IODINE

A healthy brain growth for your infant requires 220 micrograms of iodine per day. Eggs, pork, fish, and dairy products are sources of iodine.

CHLORINE

You should consume 450 mg of chlorine daily as it is essential for the brain and spinal cord development of your fetus. Additives such as milk, eggs, peanuts, and soy products are healthy additions to your diet.

VITAMIN A

Vitamin A is found in carrots, sweet potatoes, and green leafy vegetables. It aids in the development of your baby's bones and promotes the formation of healthy skin and eyes. Your daily target should be 770 mcg.

VITAMIN C

Taking 85 mg of vitamin C daily aids in the formation of strong teeth, gums, and bones.

Citrus fruits, broccoli, tomatoes, and strawberries are good sources of vitamin C.

CALCIUM D

Fortified milk, sunshine, and fatty seafood like salmon and sardines all contribute to the 600 international units of vitamin D per day that pregnant women should be consuming. Vitamin D supports healthy skin and eyesight as well as the development of your baby's bones and teeth.

VITAMIN B6

Aim for 1.9 mg of vitamin B6 every day to aid in your baby's red blood cell formation. Wholegrain cereals, bananas, pork, and beef are all excellent providers of vitamin B6.

VITAMIN B12

Among the advantages of vitamin B12 are the production of red blood cells and the upkeep and growth of your child's nervous system. Fish, chicken, meat, and milk will help you to reach the recommended 2.6 mcg per day.

FOLLIC ACID

Pregnant women especially need to take folic acid. This B vitamin promotes the growth and development of the fetus and placenta and aids in the prevention of birth abnormalities involving the brain and spine. You can reach your daily target of 600 mcg by eating peanuts, orange juice, beans, and dark green leafy vegetables. But consuming meals by alone won't get you to 600 mcg per day.

HOW CAN I ENSURE THAT I'M GETTING ENOUGH VITAMIN B12?

You should take a daily prenatal vitamin or folic acid supplement with at least 400 mcg of folic acid to ensure you are getting enough, as it might be difficult to obtain 600 mcg of folic acid from diet alone.

Take these as soon as feasible or as soon as your pregnancy is confirmed if you are planning to become pregnant. Consult your healthcare professional to find out which supplement is best for you.

FOODS TO AVOID DURING MY PREGNANCY?

Certain food-borne infections may make pregnant women more vulnerable, which could complicate the pregnancy. Foods to stay away from when pregnant include:

• Raw, unprocessed milk and soft cheeses prepared from it. These might be contaminated with Listeria, a germ that can lead to **LISTERIOSIS,** a sickness.

• Food that has passed its expiration date because bacteria can grow in it.

• Products made from raw or undercooked meat, like cold cuts and sausages. These may include bacteria like Salmonella or Listeria or parasites like **TOXOPLASMA GONDII.**

• Raw fish and shellfish due to their potential for significant bacterial and parasitic contamination.

• Fish that has a high mercury content should be avoided. This comprises the majority of fish that hunt, including king mackerel, marlin, shark, and swordfish.

• Uncooked fish that has been smoked, like smoked salmon.

• Raw sprouted grains, beans, and seeds. Ready-to-eat salads and raw sprouts (bean, alfalfa, and radish sprouts Pa) can contain harmful bacteria such as **LISTERIA, SALMONELLA AND E. COLI.**

• Liver and other organ meats; raw or undercooked eggs, which may contain Salmonella germs. Liver has a high iron level, however due of its high vitamin A concentration and possible toxicity, it is not advised for a pregnant woman to ingest liver.

HOW CAN I COOK FOODS WHILE PREGNANT SAFELY? Before eating, wash your hands with soap. After using any utensils, wash them all well. Cook the meat. Wash any raw veggies, salad greens, and fruit carefully. Store food at the right temperature. Eat it right away.

HOW MUCH MORE FOOD IS NEEDED DURING PREGNANCY? You don't need to consume any additional food throughout the first trimester of pregnancy. You will require an additional 340 calories per day during the second trimester and roughly 450 extra calories per day during the third trimester. Try to always have wholesome snacks like nuts, plain yoghurt, and fresh fruit on available to help you gain the extra energy you require. Consult your healthcare practitioner to determine a plan that suits your needs.

DURING PREGNANCY CAN I EAT A VEGAN OR VEGETARIAN DIET? It is crucial to ensure that you are getting adequate iron, zinc, calcium, and vitamins B12 and D if you are vegetarian or vegan.

CHAPTER 5

IMPORTANT ADVICE FOR IMPROVING PREGNANCY WELL-BEING

Among the crucial advice are:

- **Promoting a Positive Mentality(Mental Health Throughout Pregnancy)**

Maintaining your emotional health is essential when pregnant. Elevated emotions and mood swings might be brought on by hormonal changes and the expectation of becoming a parent. Any worry, tension, or depressive sensations must be acknowledged and dealt with. If you frequently or severely suffer from anxiety, depression, or other mental health conditions, get expert assistance. To get in touch with other expectant mothers who could be going through similar things, think about attending support groups. Practice relaxation techniques like deep breathing, meditation, or prenatal yoga. Make self-care activities that support emotional health and relaxation a priority. Some examples of these activities include taking warm baths, pursuing enjoyable hobbies, and spending quality time with loved ones.

• Dietary Guidelines For A Healthful Pregnancy

Maintaining good health during pregnancy and fetal growth depend on what you eat. Because you are feeding your developing kid as well as yourself during this time, your nutritional needs increase. Eat a diet rich in fruits, vegetables, lean protein, and whole grains in order to achieve a balanced diet. These foods supply important minerals, vitamins, and fiber. Incorporate meals high in folate, like legumes and leafy greens, to aid in the formation of the baby's neural tube. For more specific dietary recommendations suited to your requirements and any pregnancy-specific dietary restrictions or concerns, speak with your healthcare professional.

• Level Of Physical Fitness (Workouts And Getting Pregnant)

Frequent exercise during pregnancy helps ease typical discomforts like constipation and back pain, as well as promote a healthy pregnancy and reduce stress. Find out from your healthcare physician what kinds of exercises are appropriate for you to perform during your pregnancy. Prenatal yoga, swimming, and walking are examples of low-impact exercises that are usually regarded as healthy and safe. Steer clear of activities that put you at risk for abdominal trauma or falls. Pay attention to your body and adjust or cease any workout that makes you feel discomfort, lightheaded, or breathless. When working out, wear supportive footwear, loose apparel, and drink plenty of water. Always remember to properly warm up and cool down, and perform the recommended stretching exercises.

• Handling Typical Pregnancy Symptoms

Pregnant women frequently feel pain and discomfort during their pregnancy. These aches and pains can range in intensity and frequency from exhaustion and morning sickness to back pain and cramps in the legs. To find out how to take care of these discomforts, speak with your healthcare professional. For morning sickness, try eating small, frequent meals and stay away from things that make your symptoms worse. To fight weariness, drink plenty of water and get lots of sleep. To relieve back pain, adopt proper posture, sleep with supportive pillows, and think about getting a prenatal massage or doing some light exercise. Leg cramps can be eased by stretching and maintaining an active lifestyle. Depending on your unique circumstances, your healthcare practitioner might suggest further actions or therapies.

• Prenatal Care(The Secret To A Risk-Free And Healthful Conception)

In order to maintain your health and the health of your unborn child during your pregnancy, prenatal care is essential. It include routine examinations and tracking of your fetal development and health. By keeping up with prenatal visits, your doctor can evaluate your general health, track the progress of the unborn child, and handle any potential issues or complications. You can anticipate having your blood pressure taken, having your weight checked, having a urine test, and getting any necessary prenatal screenings or testing at these appointments. You can talk to your healthcare practitioner about any concerns or questions you may have throughout prenatal care.

• Recognizing Pregnancy Ultrasounds And Tests

While pregnancy tests verify a pregnancy, ultrasounds offer important insights into the growth and development of your unborn child. A pregnancy test finds out whether your blood or urine contains the hormone hCG. When a fertilized egg installs itself in the uterus, this hormone is released. Sound waves are used in ultrasounds to provide images of the developing fetus. They are able to detect multiple pregnancies, establish the gestational age, confirm the pregnancy, and spot any possible issues or anomalies. You can stay informed and involved in your baby's development if you know the importance of these tests and when to expect them throughout your pregnancy.

• **The Value Of Rest And Sleep Throughout Pregnancy**

Getting enough sleep and rest throughout pregnancy is essential for maintaining your general health and wellbeing. Prioritize getting enough good sleep as your baby grows and your body goes through major changes. Provide a cozy sleeping environment and stick to a regular sleep routine. Reducing the likelihood of problems and optimizing blood flow to the placenta can be achieved by sleeping on your side, ideally your left. To reduce discomfort, spend money on pillows and a supportive mattress. Caffeine should not be used right before bed because it can disrupt your sleep. Reduce the amount of time you spend using electronics before bed because the blue light they create can interfere with your sleep cycle. Try relaxing methods, such deep breathing exercises, a warm bath, or soothing music, if you have problems falling asleep.

- **Shifts In Emotion And Body(Accepting The Metamorphoses)**

A woman's life changes significantly both physically and emotionally during pregnancy. You can travel this path more joyously and effortlessly if you embrace these changes. Recognize that as your body grows and heals your baby, it will alter. Honor the wonder of life within you and concentrate on the advantages of being pregnant. Seek support from your family, friends, and partner by being honest and open about your feelings with them. Take part in relaxing self-care activities like reading, taking showers, doing light exercise, or engaging in your favorite pastimes. Remind yourself to treat yourself with kindness and recognize your perseverance and strength despite being pregnant.

• Creating A Bond With Your Unborn Child(Prenatal Bonding Methods)

Pregnancy-related bonding with your unborn child promotes a strong emotional bond and connection. Engage in activities that stimulate your baby's senses to begin building a stronger link between you two. Since your unborn child can hear and recognize sounds, play music for them or read loudly to them. Allow your baby to feel your touch when you place your hands on your belly and softly rub or massage it. Engage in visualization exercises by picturing your unborn child developing and flourishing inside of you. Engage your infant in conversation, sing songs, or even exchange letters. Encourage your significant other to join you in these activities that promote connection. Creating a connection prior to delivery paves the way for a caring and affectionate relationship following the baby's arrival

. • Making Knowledgeable Decisions(Selecting A Birth Plan And Healthcare Provider)

Making important decisions that will have a big impact on your pregnancy and delivery experience include selecting a healthcare provider and drafting a birth plan. Examine many local healthcare providers, get referrals from reliable sources, and contrast their offerings and approaches to treatment. Take into account elements including the provider's background, manner of speaking, and perspective on pregnancy and delivery. Arrange meetings or interviews to learn more about their procedures and assess whether their style is in line with your preferences and ideals. Make a birth plan that includes your choices for pain management, labor, and postpartum care. Talk to your healthcare practitioner about your birth plan to make sure it is feasible and to handle any possible issues or complications.

• Labor And Delivery Preparation(What To Expect)

It's critical to get ready for labor and delivery as your due date draws near. Learn to recognize the warning signs of preterm labor, which include vaginal bleeding, frequent contractions before 37 weeks, and fluid leaks. Learn the procedures that your healthcare practitioner has provided, including when to call them and when to visit the hospital. Stow away necessities like robes, toiletries, and baby supplies in a hospital bag. incorporates any particular things or choices included in your birth plan. Attending prenatal workshops or birthing education programs can also be helpful in gaining knowledge and learning coping mechanisms for labor.

Natural Remedies For Labor Pain(A Comparison Of Medical And Natural Approaches)

Pain management during childbirth is a personal decision with a range of choices. Natural approaches include heat or cold treatment, massage, breathing exercises, relaxation techniques, and hydrotherapy (using water to relieve pain, including taking a warm bath or shower). During labor, these techniques can aid with pain management and encourage relaxation. Pain relief can also be achieved by medical procedures like epidural anesthesia, analgesic drugs, or nitrous oxide. During prenatal appointments, it is crucial to go over the various pain management alternatives with your healthcare practitioner and weigh the advantages, risks, and potential implications on the course of labor. Knowing your alternatives gives you the power to decide in a way that best suits your tastes and your birth plan.

• Handling The Difficulties Of Pregnancy: High-Risk Elements And Issues

Due to a number of variables, including the mother's age, any underlying medical issues, or pregnancy-related difficulties, certain pregnancies are deemed high-risk. If you have a pre-existing medical condition or encounter any pregnancy-related issues, such as gestational diabetes, preeclampsia, or placenta previa, it is imperative that you speak with your healthcare professional. To encourage a healthy pregnancy and the best possible fetal development, your healthcare professional will create a treatment plan and regularly monitor your status. You can guarantee the best results for both you and your child by taking proactive measures to solve these obstacles.

• The Fundamentals Of Breastfeeding: Advantages, Methods, And Difficulties

There are several advantages to breastfeeding for both you and your child. It offers the best nutrition possible, strengthens the baby's immune system, fosters attachment, and aids in your postpartum recuperation. To guarantee a great nursing experience, educate yourself on breastfeeding procedures, such as appropriate latch and placement. Consult lactation experts or join a breastfeeding support group if you experience any issues latching, producing enough milk, or experiencing discomfort during nursing. Keep in mind that nursing is a skill that can be learnt and may call for persistence and repetition. If breastfeeding is not an option for you or is not feasible, speak with your healthcare professional to learn about other feeding methods and get the help you need.

• Recuperating After Childbirth: Taking Care Of Yourself

A crucial stage of postpartum healing necessitates care and attention to oneself. Prioritize your well-being to facilitate recovery and cope with the responsibilities of caring for your infant. When you can, try to get lots of rest and sleep. Consume nutrient-dense, well-balanced foods to aid in your recuperation and, if necessary, during lactation. Drink plenty of water, and think about taking any vitamins that your doctor has prescribed. Seek assistance from your family, friends, and spouse to help you with baby care and domestic chores. Keep track of your healing progress, discuss any concerns with your healthcare practitioner, and get advice on family planning and contraception by attending regular postpartum appointments.

CONCLUSION

Your pregnant journey is a special and life-changing event. You can guarantee that your pregnancy will be safe and healthy for both you and your unborn child by putting your health and mental well-being first and making wise decisions. Join groups for expectant parents, ask for help from medical professionals, and have faith in your capacity to handle the ups and downs of pregnancy. As you bring a new life into the world, embrace this amazing time and treasure the moments.